Nourishing Wisdom for Healthy Aging

H.-G. Saenger

The Book:

This book provides a comprehensive guide to healthy eating as we age, offering practical tips, research-based advice, and a holistic approach to nourishment. It is designed to help you understand the changes your body goes through as you age and how to respond to those changes with sound nutritional choices. But this is not just a book about nutrition—it's a book about aging well, staying active, and enjoying a high quality of life for years to come.

The Author:

H.-G. Saenger
passionate reader and
author with a wide range of interests,
lives since 2020 with his second wife
wife in Thailand.

Nourishing Wisdom for Healthy Aging

by

H.-G. Saenger

Dedication

For Britta and Laura

1. Edition, 2023

No.4/2 , Moo.7

A.Mueang , Ban Khok

67000 Phetchabun

H.-G. Saenger

„Tell me what you eat,
and I'll tell you who you are."

Jean-Anthelme Brillat-Savarin

Table of Contents:

Introduction: The Intersection of Aging and Nutrition

First of all, I would like to introduce myself to you and tell you about my life and why I believe that a healthy diet is very important, especially for us seniors.

Unfortunately, I didn't pay attention to my diet for a long time, I ate fast food when my stomach was growling and I always had a lot of stress and trouble at work. All this affected my stomach and I had problems with reflux, and I was also overweight and had high blood pressure. All in all, I lived and ate very unhealthily. Then, at the age of 56, I had a personal disaster. After 36 years of marriage, my wife thought that a younger man would suit her better, I was at the bottom and started drinking. If I had continued like that, I wouldn't be alive today. Fortunately I have two fantastic daughters, the eldest studied ecotrophology (nutritional sciences) and the younger one is a registered nurse. I learned a lot from both of them and followed their advice. I stopped drinking, started doing some sport and, above all, I learned to eat healthily. Today, at 67 and retired for 2 years, my health is better than ever. I now live in Thailand and have married a very lovely and kind Thai widow who shares my preference for healthy food and a healthy lifestyle. We do some sport every day and eat a lot of vegetables and fruit, which is of course much easier in Thailand than in England. When I see what grows in our garden alone, I could open a shop in England. Bananas, mango, coconuts, watermelons, papayas and noni (I'll come back to that later). But also vegetables that I didn't know from Europe. Thai cuisine is not one of the healthiest and best cuisines in the world for nothing.

As we age, our bodies change, and so do our nutritional needs. What served us in our 20s and 30s might not be the same thing that will support us in our 60s, 70s, and beyond. However, understanding what those changing needs are and how to adapt can sometimes feel overwhelming. This is where „ Nourishing Wisdom for Healthy Aging" comes in.

This book provides a comprehensive guide to healthy eating as we age, offering practical tips, research-based advice, and a holistic approach to nourishment. It is designed to help you understand the changes your body goes through as you age and how to respond to those changes with sound nutritional choices. But this is not just a book about nutrition—it's a book about aging well, staying active, and enjoying a high quality of life for years to come.

Our journey through life is not solely determined by the passing of years but by how we live those years. Nutrition plays a vital role in this journey. From supporting heart health to bone strength, managing blood sugar levels to boosting cognitive health, proper nutrition can significantly influence our overall wellbeing as we age.

Yet, there's more to healthy aging than following a diet or counting calories. It's about understanding and embracing a lifestyle that includes a balanced diet, regular exercise, proper hydration, adequate sleep, and a positive mindset. It's about appreciating food as a source of nourishment, joy, and communal celebration. It's about understanding that our nutritional needs are deeply personal and can vary widely based on factors like genetics, lifestyle, and existing health conditions.

In this book, we'll dive deep into the science of aging and nutrition, explore the nutritional needs of older adults, and provide practical advice on eating right for a healthy heart, strong bones, and a sharp mind. We'll delve into the role of hydration, the power of fiber, the importance of vitamins and minerals, and how to plan and prepare meals suitable for seniors. We'll also discuss how to eat well on a budget, learn from the nutritional habits of the longest-lived people on earth, and address common dietary concerns that come with aging.

The goal of: „Nourishing Wisdom for Healthy Aging" is to empower you with the knowledge and resources you need to make informed dietary choices and embrace a lifestyle that supports healthy aging. Whether you're an older adult wanting to enhance your health through better nutrition, a caregiver seeking to support a loved one, or simply someone preparing for the future, this book is your guide to nourishing your body and mind for a vibrant and healthy life in your golden years.

Chapter 1: The Biology of Aging: A Primer

Aging is a natural part of life, a complex process involving various biological changes that occur over time. Understanding the biology of aging is fundamental to grasp the importance of nutrition and its impact on our health as we age. In this chapter, we delve into the basics of aging biology, touching on the process's key aspects.

As we age, our cells experience a phenomenon called senescence, where they lose their ability to divide and function efficiently. Senescence can contribute to age-related diseases and the overall process of aging. While it's a natural part of life, certain factors, like oxidative stress, inflammation, and DNA damage, can accelerate the process.

Our metabolic rates also change as we age. The metabolic rate is the rate at which our bodies burn calories for energy. With age, this rate often slows down, leading to weight gain and increased fat accumulation if food intake is not adjusted accordingly. Moreover, age-related loss of muscle mass, or sarcopenia, contributes to a slower metabolic rate since muscle burns more calories than fat. Proper nutrition and regular exercise can help maintain muscle mass and a healthy metabolic rate.

Another critical aspect of aging biology is the immune system. With age, the immune response weakens, a phenomenon known as immunosenescence. This can make older adults more susceptible to infections and diseases. Adequate nutrition is vital to support immune health and help fend off illnesses.

Lastly, aging affects our gastrointestinal system. Aging can reduce our sense of taste and smell, affect our ability to chew and swallow, and slow down digestion. These changes can impact our appetite and how well we absorb nutrients from the foods we eat. Understanding these changes can help us adapt our diets and eating habits to ensure we continue to get the nutrients we need as we age.

By understanding the biology of aging, we can make informed decisions about our diet and lifestyle to support our health and wellbeing throughout our lives. In the following chapters, we'll explore how to do just that.

Chapter 2: The Nutritional Needs of Older Adults

As we age, nutritional needs may change due to a variety of factors such as decreased physical activity, altered metabolism and changes in body composition. Meeting these special nutritional needs is critical to promoting healthy ageing and preventing chronic disease in older adults. Below is some important information about the specific nutritional needs of older adults based on the information available:

Nutrient-rich diets: Older adults have similar or even higher nutritional needs than younger adults, although they require fewer calories. A nutrient-rich diet is important to ensure that they are adequately nourished while keeping their calorie intake in check. This should focus on foods that provide a large amount of essential nutrients per calorie.

Increase protein intake: Protein intake is critical for maintaining muscle mass, especially in older adults who tend to lose muscle. Many older adults do not consume enough protein, which can have a negative impact on their health. Therefore, it is recommended to use protein sources such as seafood, dairy products, fortified soy alternatives, beans, peas and lentils.

The importance of vitamin B12: Adequate intake of vitamin B12 is particularly important for older adults, as the intake of this vitamin may decrease with age. Eating foods rich in vitamin B12 or taking supplements as recommended by health professionals can help prevent deficiency.

Hydration: Adequate hydration is crucial for older people, although the feeling of thirst may decrease with age, making it more difficult for them to drink enough fluids. Appropriate beverages such as unsweetened fruit juices, low-fat or fat-free milk, fortified soy drinks and water are recommended to meet fluid and nutrient needs.

Healthy eating habits: Older adults can benefit from eating a variety of nutrient-rich foods, including fruits, vegetables, whole grains and dairy products. At the same time, they should reduce their intake of added sugars, saturated fats and sodium to promote overall health.

Considerations for chewing and swallowing difficulties: Some older people have difficulty chewing or swallowing. To accommodate these difficulties, it can be helpful to experiment with different food textures to ensure they can still enjoy their meals.

Shared meals and social support: Shared meals and social support from family and friends can have a positive impact on the nutritional well-being of older people.

Food safety: Safe food handling is important to prevent foodborne illness, which can be more serious for older people with weaker immune systems.

Access to nutrition resources: There are several government resources that support older adults to access nutritious meals. These include community meals from the DRC, food services from various food banks and municipal services, and care services from a wide range of institutions.

Cognitive health and Alzheimer's disease: For older adults, cognitive health is also an important aspect of overall wellbeing. Alzheimer's disease is a progressive brain disease that affects many adults aged 65 and older. Early detection of cognitive decline allows for better management of chronic disease and better healthcare planning. The CDC's Alzheimer's Disease and Healthy Aging Program gathers data and supports initiatives to address dementia through road maps and partnerships. The BOLD Infrastructure for Alzheimer's Act establishes centers of excellence and public health programs to enhance early detection, reduce risk, prevent hospitalizations, and support caregivers.

Chapter 3: The importance of a balanced diet

The importance of a balanced diet cannot be overstated. A balanced diet is a key component in maintaining overall health and well-being. This involves eating a variety of nutrient-dense foods from different food groups while limiting processed and low-calorie foods. Let's take a closer look at the importance of a balanced diet based on the information available:

Health benefits: A balanced diet offers many health benefits for both adults and children. For adults, it can lead to a longer lifespan, healthier skin, teeth and eyes, improved muscle and bone strength, a strengthened immune system and a lower risk of heart disease, diabetes and certain cancers [2]. A balanced diet also supports healthy pregnancies and breast-feeding, as well as better functioning of the digestive system. In children, it promotes healthy growth, brain development and supports healthy skin, teeth and eyes. It also helps strengthen the immune system, improve muscle and bone strength and achieve a healthy weight [2].

Disease prevention: One of the most important aspects of a balanced diet is that it plays an important role in preventing various diseases. With a diet rich in fruits, vegetables, whole grains and healthy sources of protein such as lean meats, fish, beans, nuts and legumes, we provide our bodies with essential vitamins, minerals, antioxidants, carbohydrates, protein and healthy fats [3]. This helps reduce the risk of chronic diseases such as heart disease, cancer, stroke and type 2 diabetes [3].

Nutrient diversity: A balanced diet ensures that we get a wide range of nutrients that are necessary for the proper functioning of our body. Fruits, vegetables, grains, dairy products and protein foods all provide important nutrients such as vitamins, minerals and other micronutrients that support various bodily functions [3]. These nutrients are important for maintaining healthy organ systems, supporting the immune system and promoting overall vitality.

Personalised nutrition: It is important to know that calorie needs and dietary requirements depend on factors such as age, gender and activity level [3]. A balanced diet can be achieved by focusing on regional and seasonal fruits and vegetables, whole grains and healthy protein sources. People with special dietary preferences or restrictions, such as vegans or people with gluten intolerance, can include suitable alternatives in their diet to achieve a balanced diet [3].

Avoid unhealthy foods: A balanced diet includes limiting the consumption of processed foods, refined grains, added sugars and alcohol [3]. These foods can contribute to weight gain, increase the risk of chronic diseases and have a negative impact on overall health. By minimising their consumption, we create a healthier lifestyle.

In summary, a balanced diet is essential for maintaining health, preventing disease and promoting overall well-being. By eating a variety of nutrient-dense foods from different food groups and keeping unhealthy options to a minimum, we can provide our bodies with the necessary nutrients they need to thrive. It is always beneficial to seek personalised advice from health professionals or dietitians to ensure that individual nutritional needs are met and to promote a healthier lifestyle.

Chapter 4: Protein-rich foods for muscle and bone maintenance.

Protein-rich foods play a critical role in maintaining and promoting muscle and bone health. They provide the essential building blocks needed for muscle repair, growth and maintenance, while also supporting bone density and strength. Based on the available information, here are some protein-rich foods that are beneficial for maintaining muscle and bone:

Fish: Fish, such as salmon and tuna, are excellent sources of high-quality protein. They also contain omega-3 fatty acids, which not only support muscle health but also contribute to bone health [3].

Skinless poultry: Chicken and turkey breasts are lean sources of protein, making them a good choice for building muscle. They also contain less saturated fat compared to other protein sources, which can be beneficial for overall health [1].

Lean meat: Lean beef such as tenderloin or sirloin is rich in protein and can help maintain and grow muscle. Including it in a balanced diet can be beneficial for people who want to build or maintain muscle mass [1].

Eggs: Eggs are a complete source of protein, meaning they contain all nine essential amino acids needed for muscle building and growth. They are also a good source of vitamin D, which supports calcium absorption for bone health [2].

Legumes: Beans and soy are plant-based sources of protein that provide a range of nutrients important for muscle maintenance and bone health. They are also rich in fibre and other micronutrients, making them a valuable addition to any diet [1].

Low-fat dairy products: Dairy products such as yoghurt and cottage cheese are excellent sources of protein and calcium, both of which are important for maintaining bone health and supporting muscle function [1]2].

Nuts: Certain nuts, such as almonds, are rich in protein and contain important nutrients for maintaining muscle and bone health. They also contain healthy fats that are beneficial for overall well-being [2].

Greek yoghurt: Greek yoghurt is a protein-rich dairy option that is particularly beneficial for muscle maintenance and recovery. It also contains probiotics that support gut health [3].

Prawn: Prawns are a low-calorie source of protein that can help build muscle and provide important nutrients such as selenium and vitamin B12 [3].

Canned salmon: Canned salmon is not only high in protein, but also an excellent source of omega-3 fatty acids, which are beneficial for both muscle and bone health [2]3].

Including a variety of these protein-rich foods in a balanced diet can help maintain muscle and promote strong, healthy bones. Remember that a balanced diet combined with regular exercise is essential for optimal muscle and bone health.

Chapter 5: The role of vitamins and minerals

As we age, the role of vitamins and minerals becomes even more important, as the body undergoes various changes and nutrient needs may be different than in younger years. Proper intake of essential vitamins and minerals is essential for maintaining the overall health and well-being of older adults. Below are some important points about the role of vitamins and minerals in old age, based on the available information:

Essential vitamins and minerals: Older adults need a number of essential vitamins and minerals for the body to function properly. These include vitamins A, C, D, E, K and the B vitamins, as well as important minerals such as iodine, fluoride, calcium, magnesium and potassium [1]. These nutrients play an important role in maintaining various bodily functions, supporting the immune system, bone health, cognition and energy metabolism.

Preferred food sources: Consuming these essential vitamins and minerals through a balanced diet is preferable to taking supplements alone [1]. A balanced diet that includes a variety of nutrient-dense foods can provide the necessary vitamins and minerals older adults need to stay healthy and active.

Recommended daily intake: The recommended daily intake of vitamins and minerals for older adults can vary, and it is important to know these guidelines. For example, the recommended daily intake for vitamin D should be about 15-20 mcg, for vitamin E about 15 mg, for folic acid about 400 mcg DFE and for vitamin K about 90-120 mcg [1]. Adequate intake of minerals such as magnesium (320-420 mg) and potassium (2,600-3,400 mg) is also important, while sodium intake should be limited to 2,300 mg (or 1,500 mg for people with high blood pressure) [1].

Possible side effects and interactions: Older adults should exercise caution when taking supplements as they may have potential side effects or interact with medications. It is advisable to consult a doctor before taking supplements to ensure safety and appropriateness for the individual's health condition [1].

Overcoming barriers to healthy eating: Older adults may face certain barriers to healthy eating, such as budget constraints, decreased appetite and difficulty chewing and swallowing. Overcoming these challenges and finding practical solutions to ensure a balanced intake of essential nutrients is important to support overall health in older age [2].

The role of multivitamins: Multivitamins can be a practical solution to address potential nutrient gaps in the diets of older adults, especially when diet alone does not meet all nutritional needs. Although the effectiveness of multivitamins in preventing disease is uncertain, studies suggest that multivitamins may help maintain memory in older people, especially those with heart disease [3]. However, multivitamins should not be considered as a substitute for a balanced diet, but rather as a supplement to ensure adequate nutrient intake.

Unusual food supplements: There are food supplements that I personally do not see as such, rather as an extraordinary gift of nature. These include certain mushrooms, vegetables and fruits that, when properly dosed and prepared, can help our bodies with many diseases, including cancer. To list them all here would go far beyond the scope of this book. Below I have listed some that I have already written a book about.

Noni: The noni tree is a plant species of the genus Morinda within the red family. The noni is the fruit of the noni tree. Not only is it said to help with inflammation and stomach ulcers, but it also helps the body with cardiovascular disease and depression. It is also said to have anti-ageing effects, reduce wrinkles and even prevent cancer. Noni roots, stem, bark, leaves, flowers and fruit are used as medicine. Especially the fruit juice is very rich in potassium. It also contains vitamin C, vitamin A and many other chemicals that can help repair damaged cells in the body and activate the immune system. More and detailed information in my book available on Amazon: https://www.amazon.co.uk/dp/B0BNTXTHCR and https://www.amazon.com/dp/B0BNTXTHCR

Black Garlic: Learn more about the history and health benefits of fermented black garlic. Fermented garlic protects our cells, intestinal flora and is considered a real booster for the immune system. And the so-called black garlic is much tastier than its appearance suggests. With its sweet plum note, it refines rice or pasta dishes and is suitable as a spice. More and detailed information in my book available on Amazon: https://www.amazon.co.uk/dp/B0BJ46CJ7Y and https://www.amazon.com/dp/B0BJ46CJ7Y

Onions: revealing the incredible power of the onion as a staple ingredient in healthy cooking and showcasing its versatility, nutritional value and unique flavour is my endeavour here. We look at the history and cultivation of onions, delve into their nutritional profile and medicinal properties, and offer a wealth of delicious and nutritious recipes that will make you see onions in a new light. More and more detailed information in my book available on Amazon: https://www.amazon.co.uk/dp/B0C1HZYFSM and https://www.amazon.com/dp/B0C1HZYFSM

Chillies: India and South East Asia are known for their fondness for spicy foods. Studies have shown that eating chillies has many health benefits for Europeans too. Chilli can lower cholesterol, protect the stomach lining and even stimulate calorie burning. Therefore, we should all reach for chilli more often to benefit from these positive effects. More and detailed information in my book available on Amazon: https://www.amazon.co.uk/dp/B0C2S9ZYNN and https://www.amazon.com/dp/B0C2S9ZYNN

Ginger: Ginger is considered a natural healing plant. The tuber has positive effects on the immune system and can help with colds, aches and pains and nausea. Healers and doctors in China and India already knew around 5000 years ago that ginger is healthy for body and mind. Since then, the tropical medicinal plant has spread all over the world and is now considered a real superfood. More and detailed information in my book, available at Amazon: https://www.amazon.co.uk/dp/B0C2SCNWHS and https://www.amazon.com/dp/B0C2SCNWHS

Aloa Vera: Scientists have now identified over 200 ingredients in aloe vera. It is important to know that the effectiveness of aloe vera is not simply due to individual ingredients, but to the extraordinary combinations of active ingredients. The mono- and polysaccharides of aloe vera (in juice and gel) have anti-inflammatory, antibacterial, antiviral, antifungal, immunosti-mulant and digestive properties. More and detailed information in my book, available from Amazon: https://www.amazon.co.uk/dp/B0C2RM913L and https://www.amazon.com/dp/B0C2RM913L

Turmeric: Turmeric has long been an integral part of Ayur-vedic medicine. In curry, „golden milk" or a ginger-turmeric tea, the yellow tuber has pain-relieving, antibacterial and anti-inflammatory effects. Turmeric is also said to prevent skin ageing and diseases such as Alzheimer's or cancer. More and detailed information in my book, available at Amazon: https://www.amazon.co.uk/dp/B0C47SW4ML and https://www.amazon.com/dp/B0C47SW4ML

Lion's mane mushroom: (Hericium erinaceus) just like other power mushrooms, the lion's mane contains a lot of minerals and trace elements, including iron, magnesium, potassium, zinc, selenium and phosphorus. Scientists have gone in search of clues. They were able to prove, for example, that the lion's mane mushroom helps improve mental performance in older people. More and detailed information in my book, available on Amazon: https://www.amazon.co.uk/dp/ B0C5KNPQVV and https://www.amazon.com/dp/ B0C5KNPQVV

Black Cumin Oil: Black cumin (Nigella sativa), often referred to as the „miracle herb", has a rich history dating back over 3000 years. It is known for its healing properties, was found in the tomb of King Tutanchamun and mentioned in the Bible. The Prophet Mohammed famously declared that black seed could cure every disease except death. Given this deep-rooted legacy, this humble plant and its oil have been the subject of numerous scientific studies confirming its therapeutic potential. More and detailed information in my book, available at Amazon: https://www.amazon.co.uk/dp/B0CCCVMX22 and https://www.amazon.com/dp/B0CCCVMX22

Now this was just a small selection of what good things nature has in store for us. It is not for nothing that they say there is a herb for everything, you just have to find it and use it consistently. Natural remedies are not pharmaceutical clubs that work immediately, you have to give them the time they need to unfold their healing power. But then you have a powerful tool against all kinds of diseases that have no negative side effects on your body.

In summary, vitamins and minerals play an important role in health and well-being as we age. Older adults should strive to eat a balanced diet rich in nutrient-rich foods to meet their specific nutritional needs. Although supplements such as multivitamins can be helpful in certain situations, they should be taken with caution and under the guidance of health professionals. Regular check-ups and individualised nutritional counselling can help ensure that older adults get the right amount of vitamins and minerals to maintain their health as they age.

Chapter 6: Calorie requirements in old age

As we age, calorie requirements can change due to a number of factors, including a decrease in metabolic rate, changes in physical activity levels and changes in body composition. Meeting adequate calorie needs is important for maintaining overall health and well-being as we age. While the information available does not directly address the calorie needs of older adults, I can provide general guidance on this topic:

Calorie requirements in older age: The calorie requirements of older adults depend on several factors, including age, gender, weight, height, physical activity and general health. In general, older adults require fewer calories than younger adults due to a lower basal metabolic rate and possibly lower activity levels. However, it is important to know that individual calorie needs can vary significantly.

Healthy eating and balanced diet: Older adults should focus on a balanced diet that includes a variety of nutrient-dense foods to meet their nutritional needs while controlling calorie intake. Emphasis should be placed on whole grains, lean protein, fruits, vegetables and healthy fats. Adequate intake of vitamins, minerals and other essential nutrients is critical for overall health and to prevent nutrient deficiencies.

Nutrition programmes and resources: Nutrition programmes and resources designed specifically for older adults can provide valuable guidance on meeting their nutritional needs. The Toolkit for Senior Nutrition Programs and resources on websites such as Nutrition.gov provide useful tips and information for older adults and their caregivers to ensure they are getting the right nutrition for their age and health status [1]2.

Dietary supplement drinks: In some cases, it can be difficult for older people to meet their calorie and nutrient needs through regular meals alone. Dietary supplement drinks may be considered under the guidance of healthcare professionals to provide additional nutrients and support overall health.

Calorie calculator: While the information provided includes a general calorie calculator, it is important to note that the calculators are usually based on general population averages and may not take into account the specific needs of older people. Individualised dietary advice from healthcare professionals, such as dietitians, may be more accurate and tailored to the individual's needs.

In summary, calorie needs can vary with age due to individual factors and it is important for older adults to eat a balanced diet that meets their nutritional needs. Advice from healthcare professionals and the use of nutrition resources for older adults can help ensure that they maintain an appropriate calorie intake and support overall health and well-being in their later years.

Chapter 7: Healthy drinks for older adults

Healthy drinks for older adults should aim to provide important nutrients while being enjoyable and easy to consume. As we age, it is important to drink enough fluids and eat right to promote overall health and well-being. Based on the available information, here are some healthy beverage options for older adults:

Nutritional drinks: Nutritional drinks for adults and seniors can be a convenient option to ensure adequate nutrient intake, especially for people with limited mobility or busy schedules. These drinks come in a variety of flavours and consistencies and offer a balance of protein, carbohydrates and sometimes fat. However, caution is advised with some of these drinks as they contain a lot of sugar. When choosing nutritional drinks, it is important to consider individual health needs and dietary habits to avoid excessive sugar intake [1].

Ready-made nutritional drinks: Nutritional drinks specially designed for older people are commercially available, such as Ensure Plus, Boost Plus and Orgain. These drinks are high in calories and contain a range of vitamins and minerals, making them suitable as meal replacements or supplements for people who lose weight unintentionally or have difficulty preparing meals [2]. It is important to choose products that seniors will enjoy and actually eat.

Healthy homemade options: Homemade nutritional drinks can be a great alternative for those who prefer organic products or have special dietary preferences. High-calorie shakes and smoothies can be made with nutrient-dense ingredients to prevent unintended weight loss and promote weight gain if needed. Tailoring these drinks to individual tastes and nutritional needs ensures that seniors find them enjoyable and beneficial [2].

Flavoured sparkling water: Flavoured sparkling water is a hydrating option with low sugar content. It is a refreshing alternative to regular water and can be a good choice for seniors who want a little flavour without the added calories [3].

Green tea: Green tea offers vitality benefits and antioxidant properties, making it a healthy drink for older adults. Its potentially positive effects on metabolism and cognitive function can have a positive impact on the overall well-being of seniors [3].

Smoothies: Smoothies are a versatile option that can be customised with a variety of nutritious ingredients. They can contain protein, healthy fats, fibre, fruits and vegetables, providing a well-rounded drink that can support seniors' nutritional needs and hydration [3].

Hibiscus tea: Hibiscus tea is known for its antioxidant properties and potential blood pressure lowering effects. It is a tasty option that can contribute to the overall health and well-being of older people [3].

Coconut water: Coconut water has a sweet and nutty taste while providing important electrolytes. It can be a hydrating and enjoyable choice for older people, especially in hot weather or after exercise [3].

Low-fat and fat-free milk: Low-fat and fat-free milk are excellent sources of calcium and other important nutrients. They can contribute to bone health and are a good source of hydration for older people [3]. Recent studies have shown that there is nothing better for dehydration than milk, as it not only restores fluid balance but also replenishes lost minerals and vitamins. Provided they are not lactose intolerant, they should make sure to consume lactose-free milk.

Kefir: Kefir, a fermented milk drink, is rich in probiotics that can support the immune system and gut health. It can be a useful addition to seniors' diets, especially to promote digestive health [3].

How healthy is lassi: Unlike smoothies, the yoghurt- or whey-based drinks keep you full for a long time thanks to their high protein content. In addition, the lactic acid bacteria and dietary fibres ensure regular digestion and support the intestinal flora.

Ayran: The Turkish variant of the yoghurt-water mixed drink is called ayran. It is only drunk as a salty variant. The base is a full-fat Turkish sheep's or cow's milk yoghurt that contains strongly acidifying bacterial cultures.

Dugh: is the name of the Iranian and Afghan variant of the drink. Dugh is also drunk rather salty, and the water used is usually carbonated. It is refined with spices such as cumin, finely chopped mint, parsley or tarragon. There is also a variant with finely diced cucumber, which gives the drink a special consistency.

In summary, healthy drinks for older people should focus on hydration and the supply of important nutrients to support overall health. Drinks such as flavoured sparkling water, green tea, smoothies and nutritious pre-prepared or homemade drinks can be excellent additions to the diet of older people, providing both hydration and essential vitamins and minerals. Ultimately, the best drinks for older people are those they enjoy and drink regularly to ensure adequate hydration and nutrition.

Chapter 8: Nutrition for special conditions and diseases

Nutrition plays a crucial role in the health and well-being of older adults, especially when it comes to managing special conditions and diseases that can occur in old age. As we age, our bodies change in many ways and the nutritional needs of older people may differ from those of younger people. Here is a comprehensive overview of dietary recommendations for older people with special conditions and diseases:

General guidelines for older adults:

Older adults have lower calorie needs but require similar or more nutrients than younger adults.

- - A healthy diet with nutrient-dense foods, including fruits, vegetables, whole grains, dairy products and lean sources of protein, is essential.
- - It is recommended to reduce added sugars, saturated fats and sodium.
- - Adequate fluid intake is important as the feeling of thirst decreases with age.
- - Alcohol should only be consumed in moderation as it affects older people more quickly and increases the risk of accidents.
- - The support of health care providers, family and friends is essential for promoting healthy eating habits.

Vitamin B12 absorption:

- - Vitamin B12 absorption may decrease with age. Therefore, health professionals may recommend supplements or fortified foods to meet the need.

Alzheimer's disease and cognitive health:

- - For older adults with Alzheimer's disease or cognitive impairment, it is important to promote brain health and early detection.
- - The CDC's Alzheimer's Disease and Healthy Aging Program gathers data and supports initiatives to address dementia through road maps and partnerships. The BOLD Infrastructure for Alzheimer's Act establishes centers of excellence and public health programs to enhance early detection, reduce risk, prevent hospitalizations, and support caregivers.
- - for persons and organisations who coordinate such services
- - for the volunteers themselves
- - to establish contacts with instructors for the training of volunteers
- - to promote exchange between the implementing organisations.

Tips for a healthy everyday life

- - If you make sure that these foods are regularly on your table, you have already done a lot to reduce your risk of Alzheimer's disease:

- - Vitamins from fruits and vegetables: enjoy them raw, for example as finger food.
- - Polyphenols from olive oil, blueberries and red grape juice also offer cell protection.
- - Omega-3 fatty acids are found in fatty fish as well as in cold-pressed rapeseed, olive and flaxseed oil. Use it cold, for example in salads.
- - Eat nuts in small quantities. They contain valuable protein building blocks, trace elements and fats.
- - Coffee and green tea also protect you with antioxidants.
- - Drink at least 1.5 litres of water per day.
- - Eat only small amounts of red meat.

Recommended nutrients:

- - A varied diet with adequate protein, potassium, calcium, vitamin D, fibre and vitamin B12 is recommended for older adults.
- - Eating seafood, dairy products, soy alternatives, beans, peas and lentils can help maintain muscle mass and overall health.

Hydration and weight management:

- - Adequate fluid intake is important and older adults should consume water, unsweetened fruit juices, low-fat milk or fortified soy drinks.
- - Maintaining a healthy weight is beneficial for overall health and chronic disease prevention.

Socialising and enjoyment:

- - Socialising at mealtimes increases enjoyment and promotes healthy eating habits.

Physical activity:

- - Regular physical activity is encouraged for older adults as part of a healthy lifestyle.

Use of nutrition resources:

- - Various government agencies such as congregate meals, SNAP, CSFP, home delivery services, and the Child and Adult Care Food Program assist older adults in accessing healthy foods.
- - Remember that each individual's nutritional needs may vary depending on health conditions, medications, and overall health. It is important that older adults consult with their health care providers or dietitians to tailor their nutrition plan to their individual needs and circumstances.

Overall, a balanced and nutritious diet combined with regular physical activity and social engagement can contribute significantly to the health and well-being of older people, even when specific conditions and diseases are present.

Chapter 9: Safety aspects of food preparation.

Cooking and reheating food at the right temperature and time kills harmful bacteria. For chicken, duck, pork and offal, make sure the core temperature reaches 75 °C and the meat is no longer pink and no clear juices are coming out. Beef and lamb steaks can be served rare if they are cooked properly on the outside. Use a thermometer to reach 75 °C for the inside. Fish and shellfish can be eaten raw, but cooking kills bacteria; freezing fish before eating kills parasites. When grilling, undercooked food and cross-contamination should be avoided, while reheated food should reach 75°C and be consumed within 2 days. Reheating food multiple times increases the risk of food poisoning.

It is important to prioritise food safety for our health. Over 200 diseases can be caused by unsafe food, affecting millions of people every day. To ensure safe food preparation, cleanliness is crucial. Wash hands thoroughly, clean surfaces and pay attention to kitchen areas to prevent the transmission of bacteria. When cooking, make sure meat is cooked at the correct temperature and use a food thermometer. Cool leftovers immediately and reheat food evenly in the microwave. Freeze and store food properly to avoid dehydration and freezer burn. By following these practices, we can protect ourselves from foodborne illness and promote a healthier eating experience.

Mafioso Al Capone's family played a surprising role in the history of food labelling when they advocated for milk labelling after a family member became ill from contaminated milk. Later, best-before dates were introduced, and in the 1970s they made their way onto store shelves. The date helps us avoid unsafe food, because even dangerous products can look and smell good. The use-by date is crucial for safety because it indicates when a food is no longer safe.

Best before date and use by date - what's the difference?

You have found a bar of chocolate with white, blotchy spots in the store cupboard - What to do? Throw it in the bin? No, the chocolate was probably just stored incorrectly and is still suitable for baking.

What does the best-before date mean?

Packaged food, with a few exceptions, must bear a best-before date (MHD). This best-before date must be clearly legible on the label. It is often found in the same field of vision as the sales description. If it is in a different place, it must be indicated where it can be found. For example, „Best before: see cover". A best-before date is not required for fresh goods such as fruit and vegetables in one piece, vinegar, salt or sugar in solid form.

According to the Food Information Regulation, the best-before date is „the date until which the food retains its specific properties under appropriate storage conditions". It thus provides guidance for the safe handling of food. Supplementary information is often given on the packaging if special storage conditions, such as temperatures, have to be observed to ensure that the best-before date is adhered to.

Can food still be eaten after the best-before date?

The best-before date is not an expiry date. It does not say that the product is spoiled after the date has passed. Consumers must check for themselves whether the food is still edible after the date has expired. Many foods can still be eaten after the best before date has expired. Muesli, for example, is usually still edible after the best-before date. If nuts are contained, they can easily become rancid. The most important thing is to store the products properly. Pasta, rice or flour can also be kept after the best-before date if they are stored correctly and in a dry place. Food that is stored for a long time is susceptible to pests and should therefore be kept in sealable containers. If the products are not stored dry enough, mould can quickly form.

It is always advisable to check the quality of food before the best-before date expires. Damaged packaging can lead to faster spoilage. However, it is still possible to consume food after the best-before date has expired.

Before disposing of food that is past its best-before date, use your senses. Check the colour of the food - is it still OK? Does it smell as expected? Is the packaging intact or bloated? Does it have the typical taste? Are there signs of mould? If you have any doubts, it is best to discard the food.

When is the use-by date indicated?

Food that is perishable must have a use-by date that is indicated as „to be consumed by...". For non-packaged food, the use-by date should be on a label next to the product. At the same time, it indicates how the food should be stored. This information can be found, for example, on minced meat, poultry meat, ready-made salads or raw milk. These foods are susceptible to the growth of germs and bacteria. For this reason, after the use-by date, there is a health risk and the food should no longer be considered safe. After the use-by date, the product must no longer be sold. You should no longer consume such products, but dispose of them.

If you are planning a trip to Asia, I would like to give you a few tips for your health. I have been living in Thailand since 2020 and have never had any problems with food. When eating street food, make sure to eat where as many locals as possible eat their food, as this is where the likelihood of food poisoning is lowest. Hygiene in these countries takes more than a little getting used to, but as I mentioned before, it has never happened to me that I got a spoiled meal.

However, the European stomach cannot always keep up with these foreign foods. Symptoms such as diarrhoea, nausea or even food poisoning can occur. This is usually because our stomach is not familiar with the unfamiliar spices, flavours, foods and harmless bacteria.

A particular danger is that treated fruit and vegetables may contain germs and impurities. Therefore, it is advisable to always peel fruit and either boil or cook vegetables. Unfortunately, salad should generally be avoided unless it is in larger restaurants with strict hygiene regulations.

Not all street food vendors are the same. It is important to remember that you often don't know how long the food has been sitting and how fresh it is. Especially with boiled or fried sausages or eggs, which are offered in the heat of Southeast Asia, the shelf life can be limited. It is therefore advisable to opt for dishes and meat that are freshly prepared in front of you. Soups that are still simmering are also usually safe to eat. In addition, it is important to pay attention to hygienic conditions. Should the cooks' hands be reasonably clean and should clean dishes be used?

In England, it is common for tap water to be drinkable and even considered healthy. You can easily fill a bottle from the tap and drink the water, even at airports. However, this is not the case in Thailand, the Philippines, Cambodia and other countries.

Even though it is not environmentally friendly, it is recommended to only drink water from completely sealed bottles in Southeast Asian countries. Even in tourist areas like Pattaya and Phuket, where water quality has improved, caution is advised. The Foreign Office recommends buying carbonated water, as it is easier to spot bottles that have already been opened.

An ice-cold drink is especially pleasant in high temperatures. But beware, there are hidden dangers: Ice cubes are often made from tap water. For Thailand, I can say that it is safe to order ice cubes, but I am not so sure about other countries in Southeast Asia.

Chapter 10: Cooking at home: Quick delicious recipes for your health.

Quick, tasty, and healthy: when you're short on time, you don't have to resort to fast food. With these tips and recipes, seniors can cook fresh and healthy lunches in a short time.

Many seniors don't feel like standing at the cooker for hours every day to prepare elaborate meals. There are many reasons for this:

- - Shopping and carrying home fresh ingredients such as potatoes and vegetables is difficult for them.
- - They have problems standing for a long time to prepare lunch.
- - They have to watch every penny and fish and meat are too expensive.
- -They don't want to cook just for themselves and eat the same dish for days.

Older people who are regularly active outdoors make a big contribution to their health and boost their appetite. Nutrition experts recommend that older people eat five small meals, served in appropriate portions. An optimal diet for seniors should include whole grains, vegetables, fruits and fresh dairy products. Occasionally, fish and meat can also be integrated into the menu to round off the diet.

Ideally, older people prepare their lunch fresh. It is even more fun if they prepare it together with others. Many supermarkets already offer a delivery service for home shopping. And as the following recipe ideas show, it doesn't take long at all to have a delicious and healthy dish on the table. You can prepare these dishes in less than an hour.

Breakfast

Porridge and berries: Put frozen or fresh berries in a slow cooker on a low heat setting. Add a small knob of butter, a portion of oatmeal and water. Cover and cook on low for several hours (or overnight). This will give the mixture the consistency of a bread and butter pudding. (Alternatively, you can simply stir a few berries into the warm oatmeal).

A hard-boiled egg as a garnish fresh fruit and a slice of wholemeal toast.

Wholemeal pancakes or waffles for extra fibre choose a brand that contains flax. Garnish them with fresh berries. You can also eat a handful of walnuts or almonds for a source of protein.

Yoghurt parfait Mix yoghurt, nuts and fruit together. This is a good combination of healthy fat, vitamin C and carbohydrates:

Power toast for healthy fat and some protein Spread peanut butter or almond butter on wholemeal toast; enjoy fresh fruit with it.

Poached egg Place the egg on the wholemeal toast and the steamed asparagus. Spread with a little butter.

Lunch

Quinoa salad Sauté chopped stir-fried vegetables (onions, peppers, mushrooms). Mix with pine nuts or pecans and cooked quinoa. Dress with Italian salad dressing. Eat fresh, warm or cold; keeps well in the fridge. It is advisable to steam or sauté vegetables in olive oil rather than boiling them, as this loses the nutrients.

Eggs and red potatoes Melt a knob of butter in a pan; cut potatoes into pieces and add to pan over medium heat. Cover and fry for 2 minutes. Then pour the scrambled eggs over the potatoes, pepper and toss until the eggs are hot. Instead of seasoning with salt, which can cause water retention and high blood pressure, use fresh herbs and spices.

Slice French fries cooked red potatoes. Heat extra virgin olive oil in a pan and fry the potatoes over medium heat. Top with the leftover vegetables and grated mature cheddar cheese. Cover and allow to steam and serve.

Southwest omelette Crack 2 eggs. Put 1 tablespoon of olive oil in a frying pan. Pour in egg mixture; add pepper jack cheese pieces and salsa or chilli sauce. When the eggs are firm, fold and serve with sliced avocado. Tip: Chilli and spices help to strengthen weakened taste buds.

Salmon wrap Place boneless, skinless canned salmon on a wholemeal wrap. Add chopped avocado, tomatoes, greens and plain yoghurt. Wrap tightly, cut in half and serve.

Dinner

Baked or grilled salmon steak Top each steak with tomatoes, sweet onions, dried or fresh basil, minced garlic and 1 tablespoon extra virgin olive oil. Wrap each piece of fish tightly in aluminium foil and place in the oven over low heat (300 degrees). When the fish is thawed, cook for about 15 minutes. The meal is ready when the fish is tender but still moist.

Lamb and potatoes (If you have some cooked red potatoes on hand, you can make quick and easy meals). Form small meatballs from minced lamb. Tear fresh basil into strips or use a pinch of dried basil. Cut pre-cooked red potatoes into small pieces. Slice a clove of garlic. Heat extra virgin olive oil in a pan. Sauté garlic and basil over medium heat for 5 minutes. Add lamb and sauté. Add potatoes; cover and cook for 10 minutes. Toss ingredients and add a pinch of ground pepper. Cook for a further 5 minutes.

Shrimp and pasta Heat a knob of butter and 1 tablespoon olive oil in a frying pan. Add chopped fresh herbs, garlic and a handful of shrimp. Toss and cook until the shrimp are done. Arrange on a bed of pasta and garnish with chopped fresh tomatoes.

Liver and fennel Sauté liver slices in a pan with extra virgin olive oil. Top with chopped fennel, onions and cabbage. Cover and sauté until the liver is tender. Serve.

Beans and rice Reheat a can of black, pinto or white beans. Serve with brown rice, oats or barley. You can also reheat the dish in a slow cooker and serve later.

Shrimp and fresh greens Sauté fresh vegetables in a pot with olive oil (again, you can buy pre-cut vegetables). Add cocktail prawns, which you can buy peeled, cooked and chilled. Serve with a salad dressing of berry vinaigrette and lime slices.

Chicken salad Sauté boneless, skinless chicken breast over medium heat in a frying pan with extra virgin olive oil. Add the salsa. Shred the chicken and store in the refrigerator to use for wraps, salad or soup.

When cooking is no longer possible: watch your elderly loved one and look for signs that they are not as skilled - or safe - in the kitchen as they used to be.

Some signs that older people need help preparing meals are: spoiled food in the fridge, an empty fridge, decreasing energy or strength when putting away and taking out dishes, a cooker top on, unsafe cutting techniques, burnt pans (signs that they have been on the cooker too long).

Some organisations that can provide help are:

Meals on Wheels: The various organisations cater to specific cultural and dietary requirements and deliver hot or frozen meals to those in need throughout the country. The drivers are also instructed to make sure that the elderly get your food safely.

Chapter 11: The importance of the social aspect of eating

A healthy diet is crucial for the overall well-being of older people, as it promotes longevity, physical health and mental freshness. It can reduce the risk of chronic diseases and improve independence in old age. In addition to nutrition, the social aspect of eating is also crucial, as sharing a meal with others increases enjoyment and improves adherence to a healthy diet. Tips for healthy eating in old age include eating plenty of fruits and vegetables, considering calcium for bone health, consuming good fats such as omega-3 fatty acids and various sources of protein for better mood and brain function.

The combination of sharing delicious and balanced meals and going for walks together supports physical and mental health. When engaged in activities with others, older people experience joy and a sense of belonging. This social participation means appreciation and is of great importance for self-esteem and psychological well-being.

Getting older people out of their loneliness by offering social participation, offering them a tasty and nutritious diet, also in community, and enabling sufficient exercise are among the most important tasks of work with older people today and in the future.

DGE Nutrition Circle

The DGE nutrition circle offers a simple and quick orientation for a health-promoting food choice. It divides the rich food offer into 7 groups.

- - Beverages" are at the centre of the DGE nutrition circle and, with a daily drinking quantity of around 1.5 litres, form the largest food group in terms of quantity.
- - Plant-based foods are in the groups „vegetables and salad", „fruit" and „cereals, cereal products and potatoes". They are the basis of a wholesome diet and provide carbohydrates, vitamins, minerals, dietary fibre and secondary plant compounds.
- - Animal foods from the group „milk and dairy products" and the group „meat, sausage, fish and eggs" supplement the daily diet in smaller portions. They provide the body with high-quality protein, vitamins and minerals.
- - In the group of „oils and fats", the quality is particularly important. Vegetable oils supply valuable unsaturated fatty acids and vitamin E.

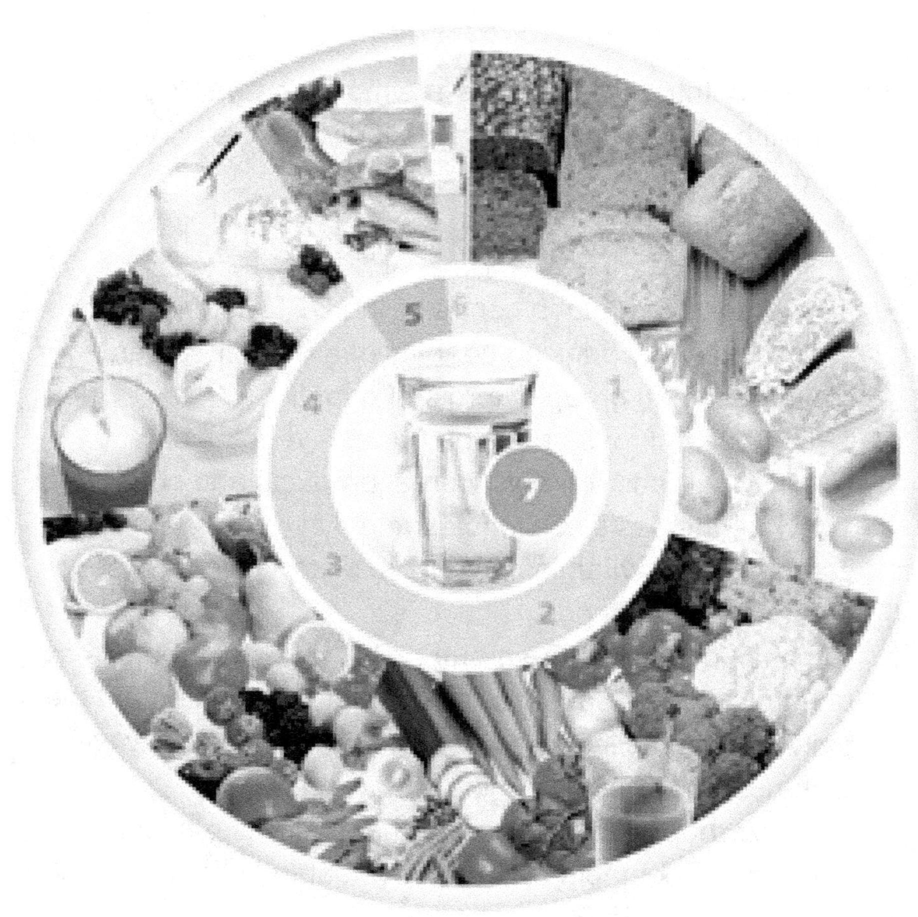
5
6
4
1
7
3
2

Chapter 12: Budget-friendly healthy foods

Foods from this category are particularly high in unsaturated fatty acids and/or folic acid, can lower cholesterol levels or keep blood vessels supple due to their special combination of nutrients. These include the following foods:

Food	Top content of	How often to eat ?	Use
Orange	Folic acid, Hesperidin	weekly 2-3 Fruits	as Snack or freshly squeezed juice
Garlic	vein-protecting allicin	at will	pasta with olive oil and lots of parsley
Por-tulaca	alpha-linolenic acid, votamin E	1x a week	as a salad with apples and rape-seed oil
Oatmeal	beta-glucans, zinc	3-4 tbsp daily	in muesli or as warm oat soup
Linseed	alpha-linolenic acid, lignans	1 tbsp. daily	in muesli, in yoghurt, sprinkled on salad

Herring	Omega-3 fatty acids, vitamin D	1x a week	Herring in tomato sauce on bread
Tuna	omega-3 fatty acids, iodine	1x a week	fried with olive oil and lemon
Olive oil	oleic acid, phy-tosterols	1-2 tbsp daily	for steaming, frying, with salad
Rape-seed oil	alpha-linolenic acid, vitamin E	daily 1-2 tbsp.	for steaming, frying, with salad
Red grape juice	antioxidant resveratrol	several times a week	as a refreshing morning drink

Beta-carotene and other pigments protect the skin from external influences and promote cell renewal. Vitamin C tightens the connective tissue, while vitamin E keeps the skin elastic.

Food	Top content of	How often to eat ?	Use
Melon	cell-protecting beta-carotene	often in season	chilled and pure, in salad, in muesli
Peppers	Vitamin C, carotenoids	often in season	in salads, with dip, steamed or roasted

Avocado	Vitamin E, B 6, Biotin	1 x a week	as Guacamole or bread spread
Tomatoes (can)	antioxidant Lypokin	1 x a week	Pasta mit with tomato sauce
Forest berries (frozen)	cell-protecting anthocyanins	several times a week	in muesli, with yoghurt or ice cream, as a drink
Apricot (dried)	Beta-caro-tene, vitamin E	3-4 pieces daily	as a snack. Impor-tant: Drink water with it

Here you will find foods that, despite their low calorie content, are rich in vitamins and minerals or satiating fibre. This makes them ideal for those who want to watch their weight but still eat healthy.

Food	Top content of	How often to eat ?	Use
Mango	Beta-caro-tene, vitamin C	often in season	as snack, with lemon juice in fruit salad
Chicory	bitter	often in season	as salad with yoghurt-honey sauce

Buttermilk	calcium, protein	2–3x a week	as a shake with mango
Turkey breast	B-Vitamins	2–3x a week	with avocado cream on wholemeal bread
Crispbread	fibre	1-2 slices daily	with low-fat herb cream cheese
Sauerkraut	fibre, mustard oils	often in season	stewed with apples, as soup
Wild rice with vegetables	complex carbohydrates	1–2x a week	sprinkled with chopped parsley
Chili	Capsaicin	at will	as a spice - even for sweets
Mineral water	various minerals	daily 1.5 to 3 litres	of still water is more digestible

Complex carbohydrates provide long-lasting satiety and have a positive effect on insulin levels. In addition, the foods contain B vitamins and magnesium, which support muscle function and provide important cell protection substances. These nutrients are especially important for athletes and are abundantly offered in our Fit Food category.

Food	Top content of	How often to eat ?	Use
Apple	Pectin, Poly-phenols	daily 1-2 fruits	grated raw with cinnamon and lemon
Rosehip	Vitamin C, Pectin	several times a week	Rosehip puree in muesli, dressing, shake
Blueber-ries	antioxidant Anthocyanins	often in season	as a shake with milk and almonds
Artichoke	Vitamin B 1, Inulin	often	cooked in season with yoghurt-garlic dip
Jacket potato	complex carbohydrates	2-3x a week	with curd cheese, linseed oil and chives
Emmen-tal	calcium, Vitamin D	2-3x a week	on bread
Whole-meal rye bread	Fibres, B vitamins	daily 2 slices	thickly sliced, thinly spread
Nut muesli	complex carbohydrates	3-4x times a week	refined with sea-sonal fruits
Millet	Magnesium, Vitamin B 6	2x a week	as a side dish with fish, tofu or meat

Kidney beans	Fibre, protein	1x a week	as a salad with tomatoes and tuna fish
Cinna-mon	polyphenols, essential oils	as desired	in goulash, with desserts, on milk foam
Pumpkin seeds	Magnesium, iron	1 tsp daily	as a snack, on salads
Vege-table juice	carotenoids, flavonoids	several times a week	as a healthy aperitif before meals

A high content of cell-protecting polyphenols, flavonoids and other secondary plant substances characterises this category. Those who consume a lot of it reduce their risk of cancer and infection and supply all cells with the optimal nutrients.

Food	Top content of	How often to eat ?	Use
Kiwi	Vitamin C	3–4x a week	as snack, chutney, jam
Broccoli	isothiocyana-tes	2–3x a week	in Asian vegetable pans, in salad
Parsley	chlorophyll, carotenoids	several times a week	as a seasoning, pesto or tabbouleh

probiotic yoghurt	probiotic bacteria	important: daily	with rosehip puree and linseed
Tofu	phytoestrogens, protein	1x a week	instead of meat or fish, in soup
Fillet of beef	zinc, iron, vitamin B 12	2x a week	in strips fried in a wok, with sesame seeds
Spinach (frozen)	carotenoids, folic acid	2x a week	with tomatoes and olive oil with pasta
Turmeric	Curcumin	at will	in curries and Asian food
Horseradish	mustard oils	1x a week	with smoked salmon, on bread
dark chocolate	antioxidant flavonoids	daily 1 bar	pure and with eyes closed!
green tea	polyphenols	daily 1-2 cups	1 tsp per cup, steep for 2 min.
Cranberry juice	Proanthocyanidins	several times a week	for prophylaxis daily 2 glasses

Back to the roots. Think back to your childhood, did you have meat or poultry every day at home? At least not in our house ! My parents had just built and my father was a simple bricklayer's assistant, so every penny had to be turned over twice. But neither my sister nor I nor my parents suffered from deficiencies, we were fed a varied and varied diet. My mother grew fruit and vegetables in her own garden and I still have the wonderful taste and smell of the delicious „across the garden" vegetable soup in my nose. There was a different dish every day and usually with fresh produce from our own garden. It was a diet that was worth watching and much healthier than what we get in the supermarket for expensive money today. Reduce your meat and poultry consumption, eat more vegetables and potatoes, you are doing your body good. This is not to say that you should become a vegetarian, God knows I'm a long way from that myself, although my eldest daughter keeps telling me how healthy it is. But it has been proven that excessive consumption of meat and poultry can cause inflammation in the body and that the nutritional value of vegetables is better for our bodies than meat. But I won't let that put me off my beloved steak, but I will cut back a bit, eat less but better quality. When I was a child, we only had a piece of meat once a week, on Sundays, two pork chops for four people. I am of the opinion that this was quite enough. Now to come back to the topic of the chapter, getting a budget-friendly meal on the table: Skip the meat and eat vegetables, you will save a lot of money.

Chapter 13: Overcoming challenges and hurdles

Proper nutrition is important for older adults to maintain overall health and quality of life, but for some it is difficult to get enough nutrients and calories. Ageing can lead to decreased appetite and altered body composition, compounded by sensory changes, depression and social isolation. Chronic illnesses, medications and dental problems can also affect eating habits and lead to unplanned weight loss and decreased energy. These barriers can be overcome through strategies such as eating a balanced diet, consuming healthy fats and fibre, and adjusting portion sizes. Problem-solving tips include using food delivery services and preparing meals in advance. Regular physical activity is crucial for maintaining muscle strength, energy levels and appetite. A healthy diet can support an active lifestyle into old age. The biggest challenge and hurdle is certainly overcoming one's inner pig dog. At least that's what it was for me, I said to myself, you can't go on like this, you have to do something and move more. So I decided to do some sport twice a week. At that time I was still in Germany and without a partner. I went to a gym and signed up. It cost me €30 a month and in the beginning I went regularly. But it was very difficult for me to get up on those days to work out. After a while, I didn't feel like it any more, but I was stuck with this annual subscription, which understandably annoyed me. Everything changed when I moved to Thailand, I was now retired and had more time for myself, and I was lucky enough to have a partner with the same interests as me. But it took us quite a while to realise that it was easiest for us to incorporate our training into a daily routine. And so now we get up every morning at 06.00 (because it gets too hot to train later in the day), drive to our training ground and train there for a good hour. There I also met an 86-year-old Thai man who is there training every day even before us. He rides his bike to the training ground every morning and does his programme, then rides a few more laps before heading home again. I sincerely hope, if I am lucky enough to reach that age, to be as fit as this man. But if I manage to keep up my exercise programme, plus the fresh meals my wife serves me every day and the most exotic fruits in between, what more could I ask for? I am now, at 67, fitter and healthier than I have ever been and I look forward to every day of my life.

You can achieve the same as me.

Go for it !!!

Chapter 14: The support of health professionals

Here you can read at three different websites what the government is planning in terms of health care and what has already been implemented.

NUMBER:1

URL: https://www.theguardian.com/society/2023/jun/29/government-aims-to-boost-nhs-with-thousands-more-doctors-and-nurses

TITLE: Government aims to boost NHS with thousands more doctors and nurses

CONTENT: The UK government plans to address the workforce gaps in NHS services by increasing the number of trained doctors and nurses. The goal is to have 10,000 medical school places by 2028, possibly reaching 15,000 by 2031. Nursing training places will also rise to 40,000 by 2028. The long-term plan aims to solve the chronic lack of frontline personnel, reduce reliance on agency staff and foreign workers. The expansion will be funded with £2.4bn over five years. Some experts welcome the plan, but there are concerns about the timing and sustainability of the funding. Labour accuses the government of adopting their policy. The NHS currently faces a significant number of vacancies, leading to worries about patient care quality. While the ambitious targets aim to meet future needs, experts emphasize the importance of improving working conditions to retain staff. The plan is expected to include measures to retain 130,000 staff members.

NUMBER:2

URL: https://healthmedia.blog.gov.uk/2023/05/25/nhs-workfor-ce-stats-for-may-2023-record-numbers-of-doctors-and-nurses-in-nhs/

TITLE: NHS workforce stats for May 2023: Record numbers of doctors and nurses in NHS

CONTENT: Record numbers of doctors and nurses are working in the NHS, helping to address the Covid backlog and provide more appointments and faster diagnoses. The NHS trusts in England have seen an increase of 53,600 staff, a 4.4% rise compared to the previous year. The government has fulfilled its commitment to recruit 26,000 more staff in primary care by March 2024, with over 29,000 additional primary care staff. The NHS is on track to meet the government's target of 50,000 nurses, with over 44,000 more nurses in March 2023 compared to September 2019. Various measures have been taken to recruit and retain health workers, including reforms to the pension system, funding for more medical school places, and support for nursing and midwifery courses. The NHS People Plan focuses on staff wellbeing, and recruitment campaigns have been launched to inspire more people to consider healthcare careers. The government aims to continue strengthening the NHS and primary care workforce to improve patient care and tackle waiting list backlogs.

NUMBER:3
URL: https://www.england.nhs.uk/2023/06/record-recruitment-and-reform-to-boost-patient-care-under-first-nhs-long-term-workforce-plan/
TITLE: NHS England » Record recruitment and reform to boost patient care under first NHS Long Term Workforce Plan
CONTENT: The NHS and UK Government have launched the Long Term Workforce Plan to address staff shortages and improve patient care. The plan focuses on recruitment, retention, and training, with a £2.4 billion investment to fund additional education places. By 2031, medical school places will double, GP and nurse training places will increase significantly. The plan aims to reduce reliance on agency staff, cut waiting lists, and strengthen the healthcare system. Healthcare leaders and organizations have shown support for the plan's ambitious goals. Emphasis is on proper funding and implementation for success in building a resilient workforce to meet future needs.

Chapter 15: Conclusion: Healthy eating as the key to a longer, healthier life.

People's nutritional needs change as they age. To stay fit and mobile, it is especially important to ensure a sufficient intake of protein, vitamin D and water.

A lack of vitamin D can weaken muscles and bones. Since our diet does not provide enough vitamin D and the skin's ability to absorb vitamin D from sunlight decreases with age, it is necessary to supplement vitamin D from the age of 65. In addition, we lose up to one third of our muscle mass as we age. To maintain it, exercise alone is not enough. We also need to eat more protein, and it is not only the amount that matters, but also the regular intake throughout the day.

While the need for calories decreases with age, the need for nutrients such as vitamins and minerals remains the same. Therefore, foods should be chosen that contain comparatively many nutrients. The motto is not to eat less, but to eat better. It should also be noted that older people tend to eat smaller and not varied meals. Social activities such as eating with friends, family or in a group can counteract this.

Ultimately, maintaining a balanced and nutritious diet in old age, coupled with sufficient social support and health care, can significantly help to promote longevity and improve quality of life.

References

NUMBER:1

URL: https://www.nutrition.gov/topics/nutrition-life-stage/older-adults

TITLE: Older Adults | Nutrition.gov

NUMBER:2

URL: https://health.gov/news/202107/nutrition-we-age-healthy-eating-dietary-guidelines

TITLE: Nutrition as We Age: Healthy Eating with the Dietary Guidelines - News & Events

NUMBER:3

URL: https://www.cdc.gov/chronicdisease/resources/publications/factsheets/promoting-health-for-older-adults.htm

TITLE: Promoting Health for Older Adults

NUMBER:1

URL: https://www.mayoclinic.org/healthy-lifestyle/nutrition-and-healthy-eating/basics/nutrition-basics/hlv-20049477

TITLE: Nutrition and healthy eating Nutrition basics

NUMBER:2

URL: https://www.cdc.gov/nutrition/resources-publications/benefits-of-healthy-eating.html

TITLE: Benefits of Healthy Eating

NUMBER:3

URL: https://www.healthline.com/health/balanced-diet

TITLE: Balanced Diet: What Is It and How to Achieve It

NUMBER:1

URL: https://health.gov/news/202107/nutrition-we-age-healthy-eating-dietary-guidelines

TITLE: Nutrition as We Age: Healthy Eating with the Dietary Guidelines - News & Events

NUMBER:2

URL: https://www.cdc.gov/chronicdisease/resources/publications/factsheets/promoting-health-for-older-adults.htm

TITLE: Promoting Health for Older Adults

NUMBER:3

URL: https://www.myplate.gov/life-stages/older-adults

TITLE: Older Adults | MyPlate

NUMBER:1

URL: https://www.amazon.com/Healthy-Aging-Lifelong-Guide-Well-Being/dp/0307277542

TITLE: Amazon.com: Healthy Aging: A Lifelong Guide to Your Well-Being: 9780307277541: Weil M.D., Andrew: Bücher

NUMBER:2

URL: https://www.nia.nih.gov/health/healthy-meal-planning-tips-older-adults

TITLE: Healthy Meal Planning: Tips for Older Adults

NUMBER:3

URL: https://health.gov/news/202107/nutrition-we-age-heal-thy-eating-dietary-guidelines

TITLE: Nutrition as We Age: Healthy Eating with the Dietary Guidelines - News & Events

Disclaimer:

The information provided in this book is for general information purposes only. The author and publisher of this book have made reasonable efforts to ensure the accuracy and completeness of the content presented. However, they make no representations or warranties, express or implied, as to the accuracy, suitability, reliability or completeness of the information.

This book is not intended to provide medical advice or to replace the advice of a qualified medical professional. Readers are advised to consult a physician before making any changes to their health regimen, especially if they have any pre-existing conditions or are taking any medications. Any reliance on the information presented in this book is solely at the reader's own risk.

The author and publisher disclaim any liability for direct, indirect, incidental or consequential damages arising out of the use of or reliance upon the contents of this book. This includes, but is not limited to, errors, omissions, inaccuracies or delays in the information provided.

The inclusion of external links or references to third party websites, products or services in this book does not constitute an endorsement or recommendation. The author and publisher have no control over the content or availability of external websites and are not responsible for the content or actions of such websites.

The views and opinions expressed in this book are solely those of the author and do not necessarily reflect the views of the publisher or any other party associated with the book.

Every effort has been made to respect copyright and intellectual property rights. If any material has been inadvertently used in this book without permission or correct attribution, please contact the publisher who will make the appropriate corrections.

Readers are encouraged to independently verify all information contained in this book and to use their own judgment in making decisions based on the content presented.

By reading this book, readers acknowledge and agree to the terms of this disclaimer. If you do not agree to these terms, please do not continue reading this book.

Other books by the author

Neanderthals: Unraveling the Secrets of Our Ancient Relatives

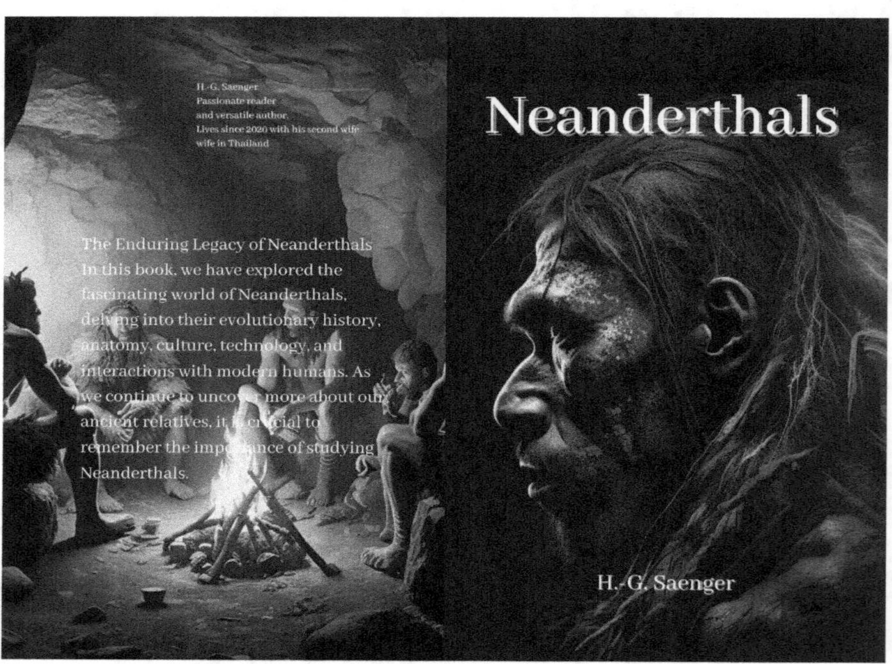

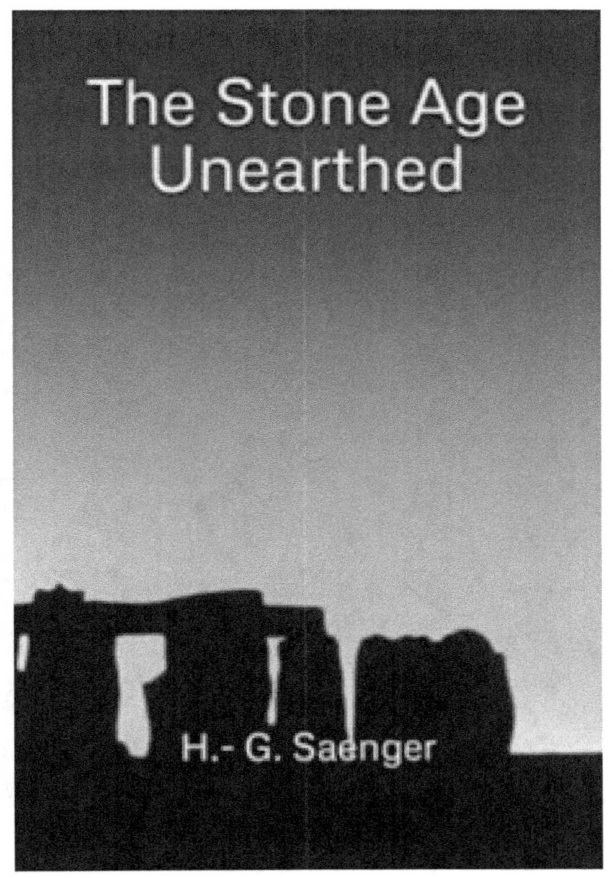

The Stone Age
Unearthed
H.- G. Saenger

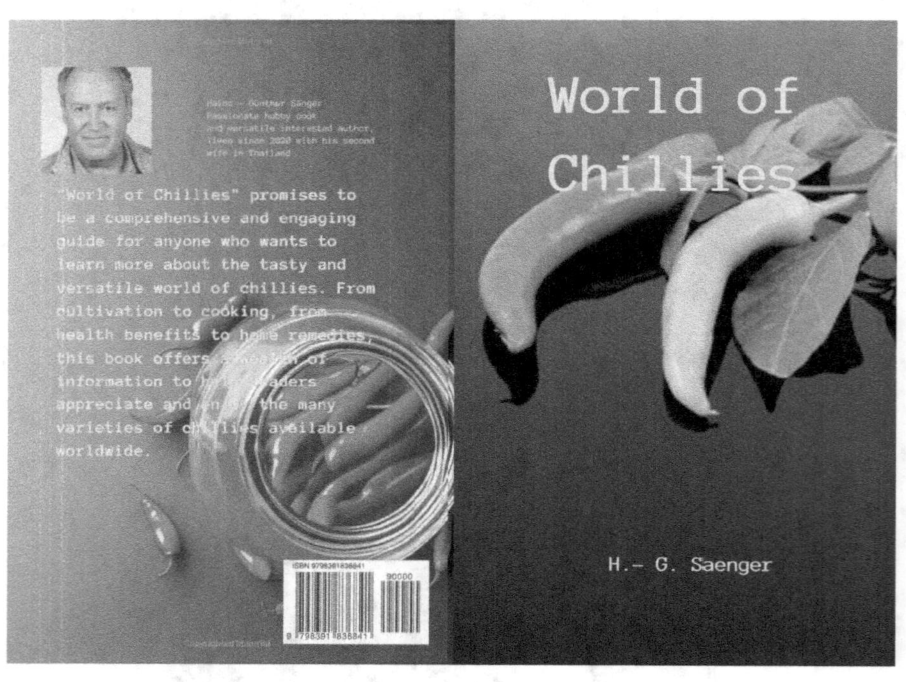
Heinz - Günther Sänger
Passionate hobby cook
and versatile interested author,
lives since 2020 with his second
wife in Thailand

"World of Chillies" promises to
be a comprehensive and engaging
guide for anyone who wants to
learn more about the tasty and
versatile world of chillies. From
cultivation to cooking, from
health benefits to home remedies,
this book offers a wealth of
information to help readers
appreciate and enjoy the many
varieties of chillies available
worldwide.

World of
Chillies

H.- G. Saenger

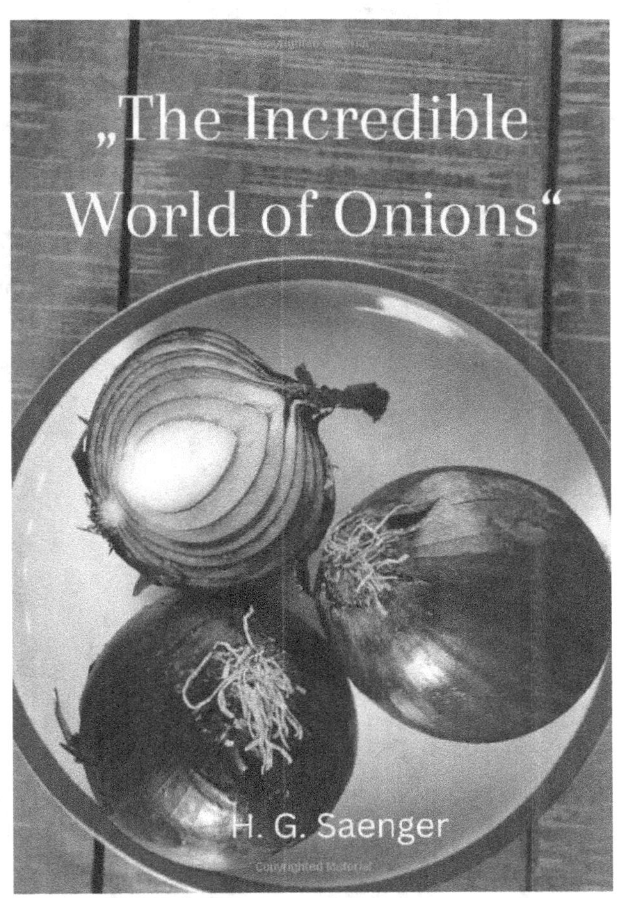

„The Incredible
World of Onions"
H. G. Saenger

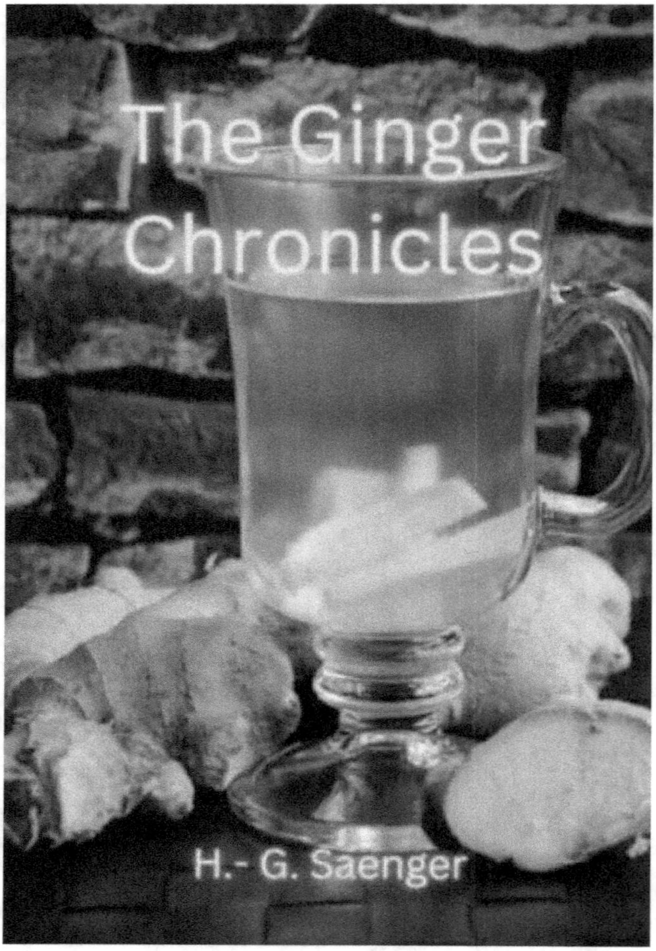

The Ginger
Chronicles
H.- G. Saenger

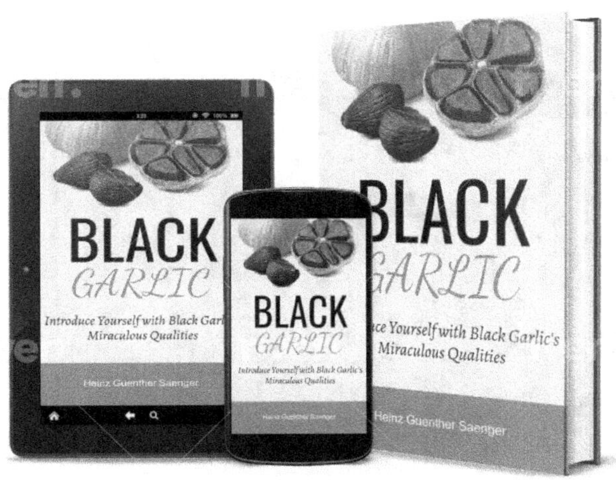
BLACK
GARLIC
Introduce Yourself with Black Garlic's
Miraculous Qualities
Heinz Guenther Saenger

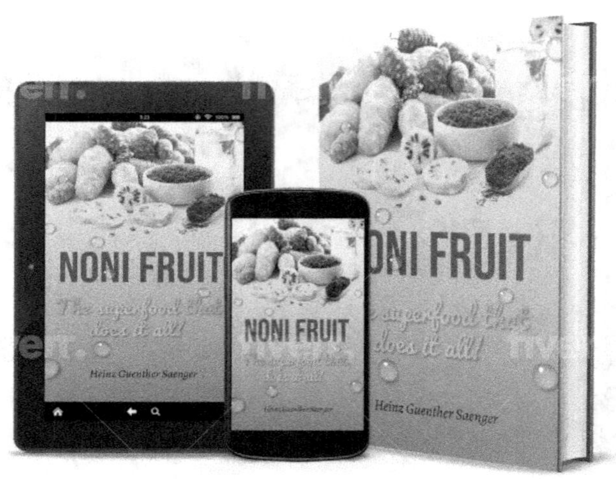

NONI FRUIT
NONI FRUIT
NONI FRUIT
Heinz Guenther Saenger
Heinz Guenther Saenger

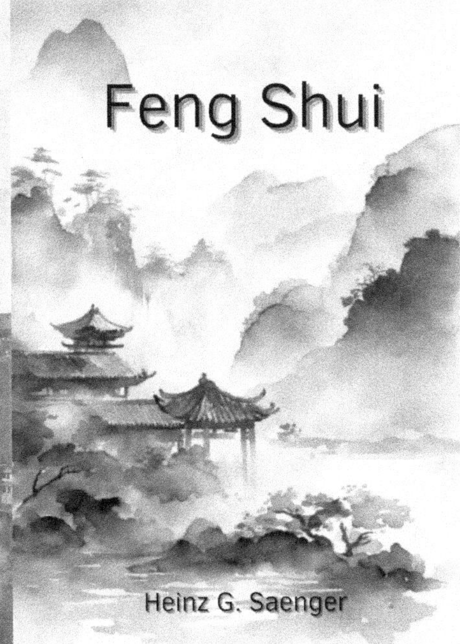
The author:
Heinz G. Saenger
Lives since 2020 with his
second wife in Thailand

"Feng Shui: Background, Meaning,
Application and Social Added Value" is a
comprehensive guide to the fascinating
world of Feng Shui. This book offers a
deep insight into the history and origin of
Feng Shui, the connection to Taoism and
the meaning of the five elements. It also
presents practical applications of Feng
Shui in architecture, design and daily life.
Discover how creating harmony and
balance in your environment can enhance
your well-being and make a positive
contribution to society and the
environment.

Feng Shui

Heinz G. Saenger

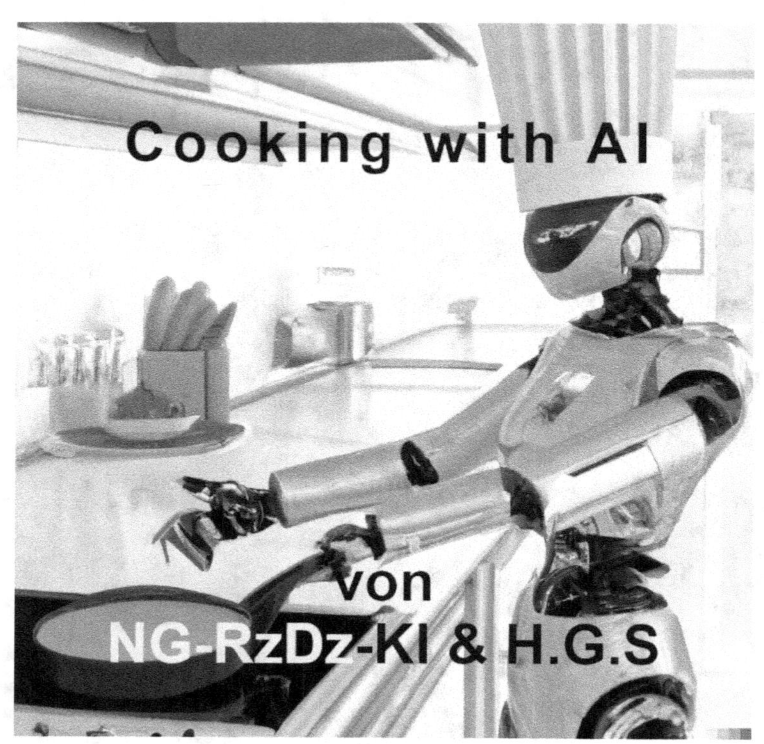

Cooking with AI
von
NG-RzDz-KI & H.G.S

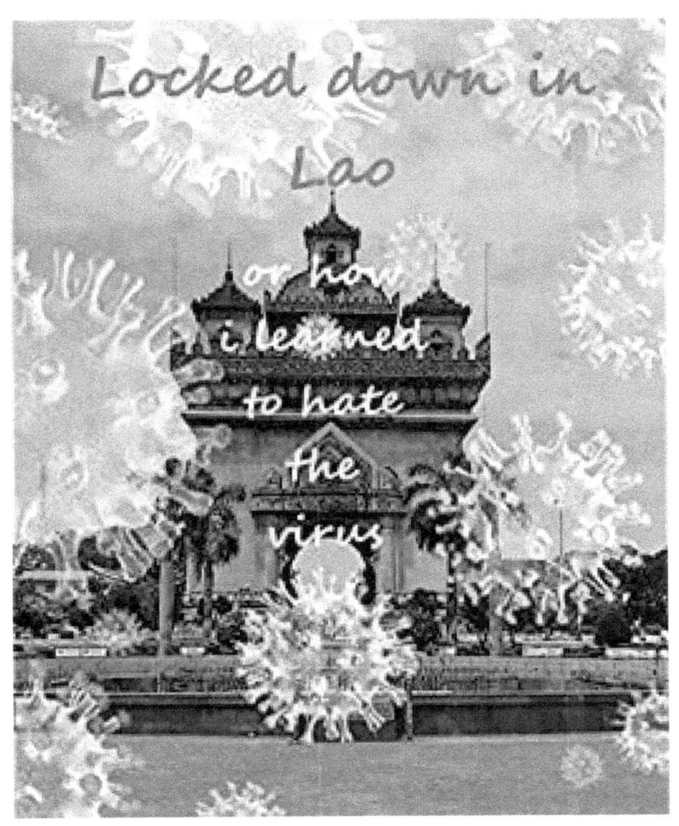
Locked down in
Lao
or how
i learned
to hate
the
virus

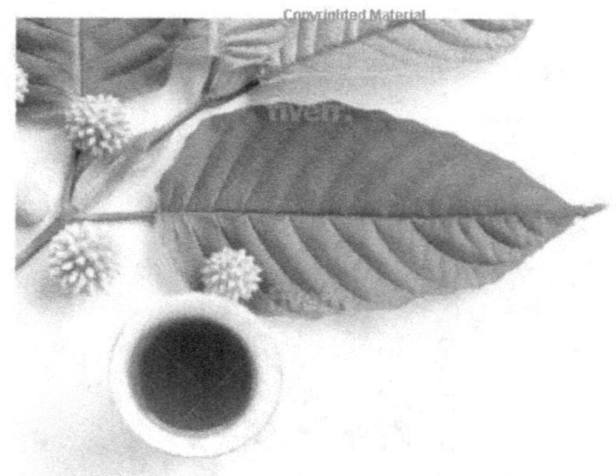

KRATOM FOR NEWBIES

All You Need To Know About Kratom Usage

By *Heinz Guenther Saenger*

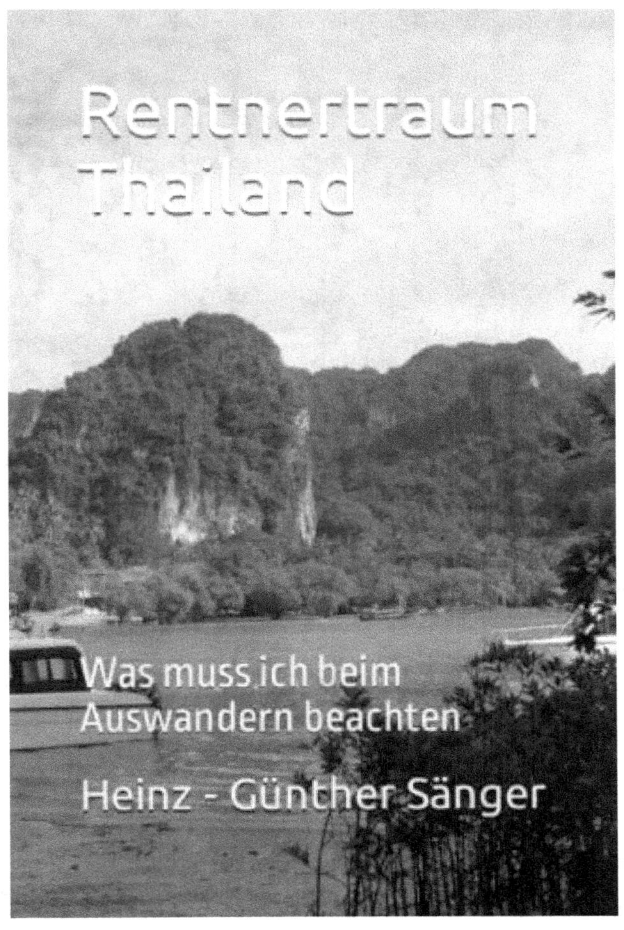
Rentnertraum
Thailand
Was muss ich beim
Auswandern beachten
Heinz - Günther Sänger

Turmeric: The Golden Treasure of Asia

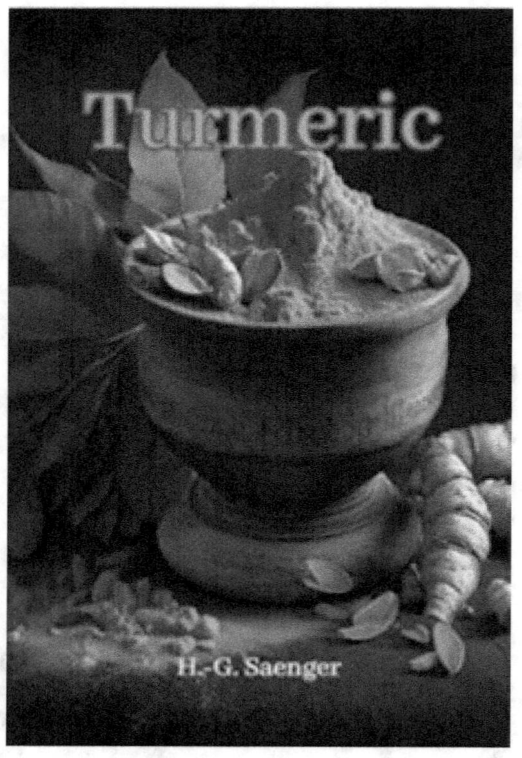

Turmeric: The Golden Treasure of Asia

H.-G. Saenger

Coconut: The remarkable world of the coconut

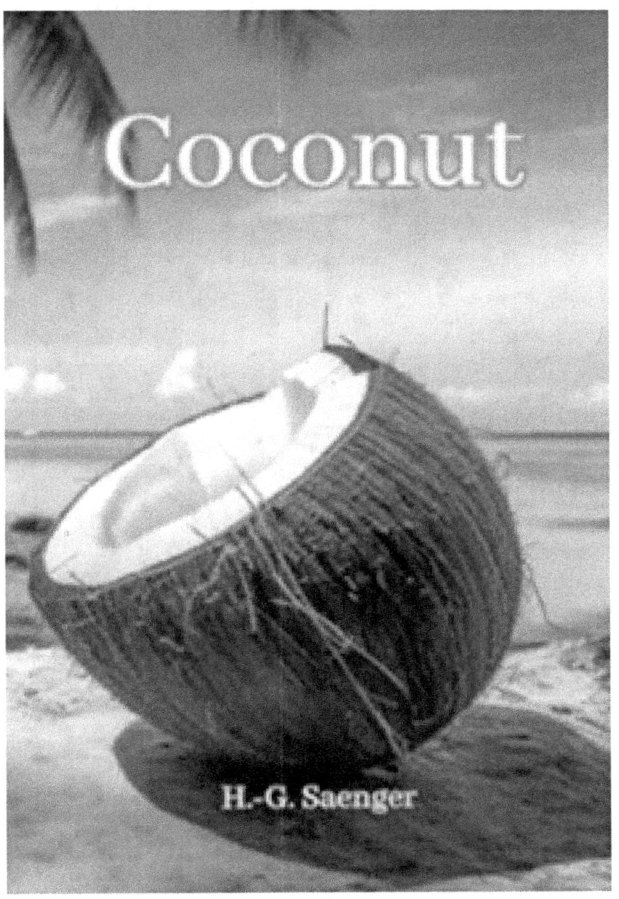

English forever: A journey through the English language

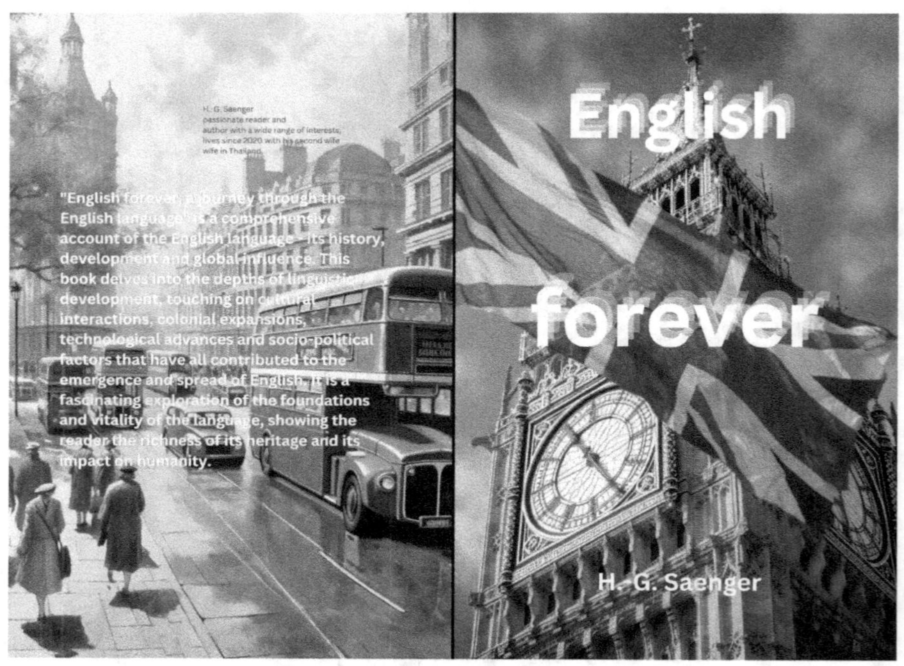

www.ingramcontent.com/pod-product-compliance
Lightning Source LLC
Chambersburg PA
CBHW070956250726
48663CB00002B/251